# THE
# CHAMPION'S
# TRIANGLE

## REVOLUTIONIZING
## PRACTICE
## IN
## SPORT

## DUSTAN LANG

The Champion's Triangle
Copyright © 2020 by Dustan Lang

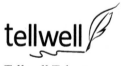

Tellwell Talent
www.tellwell.ca

ISBN
978-0-2288-3739-8 (Hardcover)
978-0-2288-3335-2 (Paperback)
978-0-2288-3336-9 (eBook)

# Table of Contents

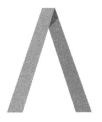

# Foreword

I am a Physical Therapist by trade with a strong passion for the health of the adolescent athlete. In my practice, more and more I am treating young teenage athletes with chronic overuse injuries. These sport injuries have many causes including poor training habits, over programming and poor practice strategies. There has been so much attention on training and over programming but not on the art of practice until now.

This book is driven from professional experience that has inspired the conception of the Champion's Triangle. The Champion's Triangle is a never-seen-before concept aimed at helping athletes, coaches, strength trainers and medical professionals. It will assist in the classification of all movements for a particular sport. This will help identify the cause of these long-standing, debilitating injuries. It can also be used as a preventative measure in designing practice in structured and unstructured environments. It can be used in an individual verses team atmosphere.

These chronic overuse injuries not only break the athlete physically, but they can also damage their competitive spirit. They are broken because they have lost their sense of self worth, sense of belonging and self-esteem. For many young athletes, sport can be their only outlet for stress and anxiety management. I have seen this lead to self-destructive behaviours such as eating disorders or cutting. It is heartbreaking to watch as a health professional. I am horrified at the immediate impact these experiences can have, as well as the implications they can have for athletes later in life.

I don't want to see this anymore. I've had enough.

I have been asked why I wanted to write a book. I've also had many people ask why I keep speaking and presenting on this topic. It's simple. I want my concept, the Champion's Triangle, to help foster empowering relationships between the athlete and sport that lasts a lifetime.

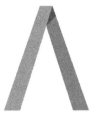

## The Telus Skins Game

The Telus Skins Game was a Canadian exhibition golf event, comprised of five PGA players, with the sole purpose of raising money for a designated charity or foundation. In 2011, I was fortunate to be selected as a physical therapist for this two-day skins format event. It was to be held at Banff Springs Golf Course located in the heart of the Canadian Rockies. I was humbled and excited to be part of this world-class event, but I had no idea it was about to change my professional life.

The event was broken up into two parts. The morning featured the pro-am side of things, while the afternoon showcased the skins match. For the pro-am, each professional started a different hole with a foursome of amateur players — together they formed a team. These teams would then compete against each other for nine holes, with the winner donating to a charitable cause on behalf of Telus. While I was waiting for one of the professionals to hit during the pro- am, a question popped into my head. How much time is actually spent swinging a club during a round of golf? I decided to spend the afternoon answering that exact question.

The skins match started in the afternoon and it was much different than the pro-am format. First, only the five professionals played, as there were no amateurs. Second, it was open to the public — resulting in a crowd of hundreds eagerly looking on during play. Last, it was on national television with an on-course host. Before the first hole, I decided to focus on one player and time him. I timed every one of his swings over the course of nine holes. At the end of his nine holes I took the total swing time and divided it by the total time for nine holes. I still remember finishing my calculation as I was walking down the back of the green. I stopped dead in my tracks.

I couldn't believe my eyes as I was looking at the final number.

It was 3%. If you put that in perspective, 3% of a round lasting four hours and 15 minutes would be eight minutes. How could that be? How could the main athletic move for a sport only be 3% when it typically produces overuse injuries? After a bit of brief work in the locker room, the players went to their corporate engagements and I went back to my hotel room. All I wanted to do was to put some sense to what I calculated earlier. I sat at my desk for hours writing, trying to figure out the rest of the 97%. That night began the lengthy process of developing the Champion's Triangle. It consists of the scoring skill, the transitional skill and the hidden habits. Athletes, coaches, medical professionals and strength trainers can utilize this tool. Down below is an illustration. The reason I wanted to use an illustration was to emphasize there are strength in the corners where the sides intersect and identical sides indicating they all contribute equally. The vision of this triangle is to help foster empowering relationships between the athlete and sport that lasts a lifetime.

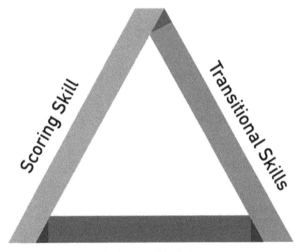

**Hidden Habits**

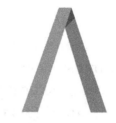

## The Scoring Skill

The scoring skill is simply defined. It is the skill set that determines the outcome for a specific sport. In golf that is striking a golf ball. For basketball it is shooting the ball into the hoop. In hockey it is shooting the puck into the net. Without the scoring skill there is no definite winner in a competitive game. One thing I have learned after working with so many athletes is that they love to practice the scoring skill. They love it — not just because they enjoy improving a specific skill set, but because they love to dream. They love to imagine performing at the greatest level and achieving the highest goals. They love to dream of creating those perfect moments that are unforgettable and inspirational. We, as sports fans, also love the scoring skill because it provides those iconic sport moments we crave. Those moments that last a lifetime and we talk about over and over. Sidney Crosby scoring the overtime goal in the Gold Medal Game at the 2010 Winter Olympic Games is a great example of this. The Toronto

Raptors winning Game 7 against the Philadelphia 76ers on a last-second shot by Kawhi Leonard in the NBA playoffs is another. Maybe the greatest of all is Tiger Woods holing an improbable chip on Hole 16 in a dramatic fashion at Augusta National on his way to win the Masters. Sports fans don't watch games just to see who wins, they tune in hoping to witness inspirational moments.

When an athlete is inspired to practice the scoring skill, they will dream during that practice session. Sometimes they can be lost in time practicing for hours. This could lead to an overuse injury as they are doing the same thing over and over. With golf, it is not uncommon for athletes to hit over 1,000 balls every day. If you break down an actual scoring round of PGA players, they will only strike the ball (driver and irons) below fifty times for a round. So why does that player need to strike so many balls during one practice session? The only reason I can think of is the will to get better and the love of dreaming. However there has to be a safer way regarding prevention of injuries. If we take a look at basketball, most players love practicing the jump shot. If you look closer, you will discover a pattern. They will tend to practice this shot from a similar distance, angle and speed of execution. I like to call it "the comfort area". Athletes prefer "the comfort area" because of previous success. When they dream, obviously they are dreaming to succeed, so it makes sense why they chose how and where they take a shot on the court. These same variables will produce repeated patterns increasing the probability of an overuse injury.

It is essential that athletes in all sports understand the importance of adding variability and authenticity when practicing the scoring skill. Variability during practice will produce a versatile athlete regarding skill development and injury prevention.

Let me explain.

If the athlete identifies and understands the obstacles for the scoring skill, then the athlete can train to overcome those barriers in a variety of situations. Let us take a look at a quarterback in football. If that quarterback repeatedly practices the same throw to the same target with the same velocity and trajectory, that quarterback is performing the same movement over and over — thus possibly leading to an overuse injury. Plus, what happens when that quarterback is asked to throw the ball in a game situation that requires a throw that hasn't been practiced? Chances are the play will not be successful and possibly predisposing the quarterback to a traumatic injury — as the athlete has not been in that position before and thus doesn't know how to handle it physically. Instead, what if that quarterback understood the importance of throwing while running to the left, right and changing distance, velocity and trajectory? This variability will utilize a variety of movement patterns, thus developing the skill set and reducing the chance of an overuse injury. More importantly these variations are authentic to the sport as there are infinite situations where the athlete must perform the scoring skill. No matter the sport, the scoring skill will never be the only skill set needed to perform at the highest level. There is always more. The transitional skills and hidden habits will always be present. It is imperative that athletes, coaches, medical professionals and strength trainers always look beyond the scoring skill for enhancing performance and injury prevention.

I want the athlete to always have the opportunity to dream while practicing the scoring skill. I want this for several reasons. I believe this will help foster the love of the game. Sometimes that love is dampened or extinguished by outside and internal pressures that are associated with playing the same sport year after year. When that love is gone, it is difficult for the athlete to fully dedicate an effort that will lead to self-improvement and team success. It may lead to disengagement from sport and physical activity, creating a very unhealthy lifestyle. Dreaming will also lead to creativity during practice. Imagining new ways to improve and succeed in game situations. This is so important for player and game evolvement. New skill sets inspire players, changes coaching strategies and modifies training and rehab philosophies. Dreaming will also continue to produce those iconic memorable moments that we as sports fans crave. Selfishly, I can't get enough of those times. Those moments are inspiring, thrilling and create an emotional moment that is imprinted on your soul for a lifetime.

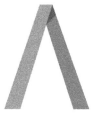

## The Transitional Skills

The transitional skills are simple — it's the skill set that allows an athlete to set up the scoring skill. In golf it is walking, squatting, reaching and lunging. For basketball it is running, jumping, landing, pivoting, passing and dribbling. In hockey it is skating, turning, stopping, passing and checking. Athletes do not typically love practicing the transitional skills as much as the scoring skill. It is not because they don't want to improve. In their mind, the transitional skills typically do not produce those unforgettable moments. However the transitional skills play a very important role in the execution of the scoring skill. If the transitional skills are performed well, this will lead to increased frequency and quality scoring skill opportunities. Without the transitional skills, the scoring skill can never be executed.

When an athlete performs any type of practice it is impossible to leave out the transitional skills. Just imagine a basketball player practicing the jump shot without dribbling. It doesn't happen. I think many times people just forget about the transitional skills and underestimate their value. But they are very important. Imagine if LeBron James couldn't run as fast, jump as high, or transition from one direction to another. The result would be fewer chances for the scoring skill or baskets — meaning scoring less, winning less and a smaller impact on the outcome of the game. If you look closely at these superstars of sport, they possess an incredible ability to perform the transitional skills of at a very high level and with great versatility. When I refer to versatility, I am referring to the athlete's ability to perform a desired task in multiple ways. For example, let us take a look at a lunge. It could be performed at multiple depths, speeds and directions. If the athlete is able to perform this activity with these different variations, then they are versatile. If they become versatile in a number of transitional skills for their sport, imagine the possibilities and movement formulas. Increased transitional skill versatility will lead to an increase in scoring skill opportunities.

Another objective of the transitional skills is injury prevention. Overuse injuries are caused by repeatedly performing the same task the exact same pattern. This includes speed, direction, depth and other variables. If we add in variations, the body will have a lower chance of being overloaded or fatigued by a repetitive motion. Changing direction and/or speed will allow the body to be stressed in a new way — allowing it to recover from the previous pattern.

There are two different scenarios in which the transitional skills are performed. The first is when the athlete initiates the movement in a sequential pattern. An example would be a basketball player dribbling the ball up the court. The player will determine how fast and which direction to dribble. Typically, in these situations, the athlete will pick their most efficient patterns of motion to yield the greatest chance of success for the scoring skill. The second scenario is when the movement is dictated to the athlete. Looking at basketball again, the defender would have to match the movement of the offensive player. This is much more difficult than being the offensive player. The reason is the defender's movement is dictated to them. Meaning the defender will have to match the unpredictable movement pattern of the opponent. That opponent likely will move to their most efficient pattern therefore creating a significant challenge for the defender.

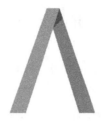

## The Hidden Habits

On the second day of the Telus Skins Game, I decided to look at things differently. I spent the first day determining a golfer will spend roughly 3% of a round swinging a golf club. Day two's focus was on what the golfer did when not swinging a golf club. There were two patterns that are worth mentioning.

I noticed one golfer would lunge and reach with the same side of their body every time they reached to tee up the ball, remove the tee, remove ball marker and pick the ball out of the hole. He did this on average of four times per hole. Over 18 holes, that averages out to be 72 times. Now if he played a full tournament — excluding pro-am and practice rounds — that would add up to 288 times over four rounds. If he played four tournaments in a row, the golfer would be looking at 1,152 lunge reaches with the same side of the body.

The second thing I noticed is the player would stand one leg crossed over the other leaning on a bag or putter while waiting for opponent to hit. This is a very common posture not only on the professional tours, but also at the local courses. Looking at this posture closely, the player is really only standing on one leg. The amount of body weight transmitted through the crossed leg is quite minimal. He adopted this posture for roughly five minutes per hole. For a round of 18, that equals 90 minutes standing on one leg while resting the other. Now if he played a full tournament — excluding pro-am and practice rounds — that would add up to six hours over four rounds. Playing four tournaments would mean that player spent 24 hours, an entire day, in that posture.

Here is the most interesting part. That player will be seen by millions of television viewers. They will golf in front of hundreds of thousands of patrons live — yet no one will really recognize what he is doing, let alone how he is doing it. That is the brilliance and beauty of the hidden habits. They convince most of the world they don't exist and the people who do see them they don't matter. But they do. Do you think lunging and reaching with the same side of the body over 1,152 times over four weeks could cause issue? What about standing on one leg for 24 hours over four weeks?

Of course!

They can lead to fatigue, muscle tightness, joint stiffness, pain, and possible injury. Here is the sad part. If that player then seeks medical attention I bet the first thing that is scrutinized, broken down and ripped apart will be the scoring skill. With our golf example, they will analyze every aspect of the swing to look for problems — when it likely had nothing to do with the injury.

One of the biggest challenges for athletes is to identify their own hidden habits. We are all creatures of habit and our bodies will always take the path of least resistance. Most times the path of least resistance is the wrong, or least efficient path. Many times these hidden habits go undetected or unnoticed, allowing them to build and impact the efficiency of the transitional skills and scoring skill. This can cause a decrease in performance and/or development of an overuse injury. The danger is then the athlete or coach attempt to "correct" the scoring skill because they believe it is the origin and not the result. What can happen is the athlete never regains the scoring skill efficiency and the injury continues because the hidden habits were never acknowledged as the source.

I believe the best way for the athlete to rid of or minimize the impact of the hidden habits is to closely monitor practice habits. The athlete would need self-discipline to emphasize variability in practicing the scoring skill in an unstructured environment. This variability will force the athlete to practice the scoring skill in different situations. This will help reduce the possibility of developing an overuse injury because there is variation in movement.

The coach can minimize the impact of hidden habits by drill design. A practice structure emphasizing a variation of transitional skills will create versatility and minimizing the chance of a repetitive strain injury or traumatic injury.

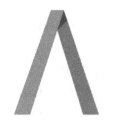

# Action Time

Following the Telus Skins game I began to think about how much time athletes actually spent playing in different sports. I will refer to this playing time as "action time". Is golf an exception to the norm? Do any other sports have a low percentage of action time? For many sports there are stoppages in play that break up the play and specific action time.

In 2010 the *Wall Street Journal* published an article, (An average NFL Game: more than just 100 commercials and just 11 minutes of play), examining this possibility for different sports.

This article analyzed the amount of action time during a National Football League game. It is so hard to believe but the publication reported an average NFL play lasts approximately four seconds. They report if roughly the hundred commercials, TV timeouts and time changing of personnel between plays are removed — only 11 minutes of action time remain.

How can a professional football game that lasts three hours and twelve minutes produce only 11 minutes of action time?

That equates to 5.72% of action time. According to ESPN, an average NFL career is 3.3 years in length. I realize traumatic injuries have a significant impact on this statistic, but how can a game lasting 11 minutes in action time produce such a short average career length.

The *Wall Street Journal* also examined the sport of tennis. Tennis is a very demanding sport physically with many stoppages in play. The *Journal* calculated for an average three-hour tennis match, there was roughly 31 minutes and 30 seconds of action time. That equates to 17.5% of action time. This number is puzzling because 30 minutes of exercise really doesn't seem very much for a professional athlete. However, if you ever watch a professional tennis match you appreciate the intensity, hard work and determination that are displayed by both athletes in every match. Players are pushed to the brink of exhaustion and injury over and over. They inspire sporting fans with the valiant efforts of an underdog or epic comeback. Hard to believe all this happens in roughly 30 minutes.

The *Wall Street Journal* also took a look at a Major League Baseball game. If there is any sport comprised of numerous stoppages of play — it's baseball. The publication calculated that an average three-hour game was 17 minutes and 58 seconds of action time. That equates to 10% of action time. Why are there so many overuse injuries in baseball? Why are there so many missed games due to injury when the action time is just short of 18 minutes? Why are some pitchers, who only pitch on selected days, stricken with life-long shoulder injuries?

What does this mean?

Simply, this means our athletes are not developing chronic overuse injuries due to competing. It isn't possible. The numbers are too low. If it isn't due to actual competition what is the cause?

Simple — it's us.

I say 'us' meaning athletes, coaches, strength trainers and medical professionals.

It is our methods of practice. It is how we self practice. It is how we design practices. Our philosophy of practice-more is better. The mindset of our workout programs cause problems, as does no pain, no gain rehab sessions. Something is wrong and philosophies need to be re-examined.

I want to explore the design of practice for the sake of skill enhancement and for the prevention of overuse and traumatic injuries.

We are missing something.

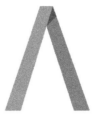

# Misconceptions of Practice

Practice is an art and science all in one. There are many thoughts, philosophies and beliefs incorporated in various sports, skill sets and age groups. Athletes, parents, strength trainers, coaches and medical professionals continuously scrutinize these philosophies and designs. Theories and concepts evolve over time, with the hope of advancing skill development and prevention of injury. With all these changes and advancement, there continues to be misconceptions regarding the design and implementation of practice.

If you look at most sports over the past twenty years, the season of play has dramatically increased. For instance, hockey traditionally ran throughout the winter months — now there is spring and summer hockey. The volleyball season typically was during the fall but now runs throughout winter and into spring. Basketball initially ran only during the winter months but now is included during the springtime. Why is this happening and why are players committing to these excessive regimes?

It's simple — fear.

Fear the athlete will fall behind their competitors and teammates. Fear the athlete won't reach their full potential. There are many dangers with this belief.

These extended seasons may impact the athlete by suffocating the love of competition and the process of getting better. Remember, all athletes love to dream during scoring skill practice and if this love is impacted, the athlete will not want to practice anymore. The athlete may also experience excess fatigue resulting in sloppy transitional and scoring skills, increased hidden habits and overuse/traumatic injuries.

Another misconception is rest will impede skill devlopment. It's one of the most important aspects for an athlete and yet it is continuously neglected — especially when talking about adolescent athletes. Practices are scheduled prior to school or very late in the day, compromising the athlete's sleep routine. A lack of rest affects the athlete's ability to perform in competition, handle the physical vigor of practice and the mental stresses of life. Plus, how is an athlete able to fully recover from the stress of exercise without sufficient sleep? A tired and unrested athlete is not a happy, healthy athlete. An athlete needs the opportunity to rest and recharge to meet the demands of sport and everyday life.

Early specialization is a problem with many sports. There is a misconception only an athlete who specializes early will reach their full potential. Playing a variety of sports will develop a variety of skill sets — thus developing a more versatile athlete compared to one who specializes early. We also see athletes who specialize early lose their love of sport and they will tend to disengage from practice. These athletes are then prone to suffer overuse or chronic injuries, because specializing repeatedly overloads the body in specific patterns of movement. The body will tend to break down when performing the same action in a repetitive fashion.

Duration and frequency of practice has significantly increased for many sports. A misconception many people believe is, "more is better."

Meaning the more an athlete practices, the greater the skill development and individual success as an athlete. However, the importance and value of rest days within the competitive season is completely disregarded. Proper rest and recovery is disregarded and ignored. Instead the emphasis is placed on trying to get the athlete practicing more. The increased workload can overload the body and increase the chance of injury.

Another misconception is that athletes need never-ending conditioning. Meaning they need to be worked extremely hard at practice — every practice. Coaches and trainers work them so hard they are very sore and fatigued following. The problem is, when you carry out this mindset the exercise is typically very repetitive with little to no variation. As a result the athlete is prone to developing a repetitive strain injury. There is a risk with this strategy. The athlete may actually decondition because of excessive physical stress and insufficient recovery time due to increased practice time.

There is belief practicing the team's systemic pattern of attack will make the athlete stronger and better suited to handle competitive play. This approach is typically carried out in an artificial environment. Meaning it isn't sport-specific. An example of this is a hockey team working on breaking out of their zone over and over with no pressure from a simulated opponent. In this situation the athletes choose how and when to move. This isn't authentic to hockey. These players will face pressure from opponents in an unpredictable way, thus influencing decision of movement in a spontaneous fashion. If the team doesn't add the spontaneous element, then the practice is artificial. An artificial practice will not prepare the team for the spontaneous moments that typically occur in real game situations.

There are more misconceptions but I just wanted to share a few. I believe most times the decisions regarding these misconceptions were for the benefit of the athlete. The heart was in the right place but unfortunately it does not produce the response in the best interest of the athlete.

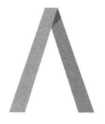

# Versatility

The word versatility has been used extensively in this book. What is it? Why is it important? How do you achieve it?

I believe versatility, pertaining to movement, describes the ability to function in a variety of ways for a specific task. For example, let us look at dribbling a ball in soccer. An athlete may choose to dribble always to the right with the same speed when approached by a defender. That isn't versatility. That is repetitive. It is a habit and possibly could develop into a hidden habit. If our athlete would dribble in many directions with various speeds, that would demonstrate versatility. Another example would be that same soccer player only passing or shooting with their dominant leg. Suddenly that athlete may be limited to movement patterns only using one side. By emphasizing both sides of the body, this will increase the movement patterns associated with shooting or passing — plus transitioning in and out of these skill sets. Sometimes the mechanical components of one type of skill will assist in the formation of another. Take for example, kicking a ball. The plant leg during that execution is also present when planting and changing direction while running. That is the power of placing importance on versatility. It fosters skill development in multiple ways.

Versatility is the most important characteristic an athlete can possess regarding enhancing performance and avoiding overuse injuries. One of the biggest challenges an athlete faces is reading and reacting to an opponent's unpredictable movement. It is difficult because the athlete does not know when or where the next movement will take place. It is dictated to the athlete. They don't always get to decide when, how and where they move. If the athlete is not versatile, then it will be difficult to follow and interact appropriately. When the body is presented with an unpredictable situation and has to read and react, it will resort to what is most familiar. Therefore it is important to develop versatility so the body will have many options to choose from when encountering that situation. If not, the body will just resort to the same familiar pattern repeatedly — leading to an eventual overuse injury.

Movement variation can help the athlete adapt to spontaneous or unpredictable situations often presented in sport. If a soccer player only practices dribbling to the right, then that athlete will default to that same strategy when pressured by an opponent. Because that is what the body knows best. However, if that same athlete would practice dribbling with variation of direction and speed, then there would be a multiple of choices when pressured. Multiple variations of motion nurtures further skill development because the body is able to perform more actions. As the skill set increases, so does the ability to become versatile. They build off one another.

Sometimes in sport, an athlete's sporting demands are very specific. As I have mentioned, the golf swing is repetitive and specific. These characteristics can lead to an overuse injury. This athlete could practice different movement variations to create variability since the scoring skill (golf swing) in this instance will not. In this scenario, the athlete could train the transitional skills emphasizing variation to encourage versatility. Versatility will allow the body to be much more tolerant of rigid repetitive motion since the body is able to move in multiple directions.

I calculated that the transitional skills in golf account for 97% of all movements within a round. It makes sense for the athlete to train the transitional skills with variation to increase versatility of the overall skill set. This is a unique but incredibly effective strategy. Think about it for a minute. The scoring skill in golf is specific but maybe the coach doesn't want variation of motion when practicing the scoring skill. Maybe the coach is concerned that if the athlete creates scoring skill variation, it could impact the overall efficiency of the scoring skill. Maybe the coach is very particular about how the athlete executes the golf swing. It is important to consider training the transitional skills with variation in order to improve efficiency of those skills. Sometimes this can have a positive impact indirectly on the scoring skill. This would enable the scoring skill to withstand repetitive motion without changing scoring skill technique.

For instance, the hip movement used in golf's backswing is required for walking. There is a strong possibility that enhancing this hip motion intended for walking will foster and nurture an efficient backswing. However, the opposite is also a possibility. An inefficient walking pattern could negatively impact the golf backswing. It is then possible the athlete could variably train the hip motion pertinent to walking and prevent those inefficient patterns regarding walking and the golf swing. If the athlete presents with a hip injury and is unable to swing a golf club due to pain, treatment could focus on the transitional skills. A movement-based treatment approach could incorporate movement exercises replicating the functional demands for walking. Not only could the exercises be corrective in nature but also emphasize versatility for that specific task. This approach would have positive effects for the golf swing — possibly resolving pain and improving overall performance of the golf backswing.

How do you create versatility? Simply through practice design. Practice with emphasis on loading the nervous system. By "loading" I don't mean introducing heavy weights like in strength training. The nervous system can be loaded by introducing different movement patterns at different speeds or directions. This loading will force the nervous system to take inventory of what movement is required at that moment. It will then compare the requirement to what the body's capabilities are.

The nervous system is like the computer for the body. It regulates all bodily functions including formulating patterns of motion. How does the nervous system do that? It does so by meeting the demands that are presented and encountered. The body takes notice of these challenges and adapts by improving movement abilities. This allows the body to overcome these demands if presented with the same situation again. It is important the nervous system is continually presented with variation of movement. This not only fosters movement versatility but efficiency as well. This efficiency will provide choices when the body encounters an unpredictable situation. It will provide choices because the body will trust it at this point. If the body trusts it, then it will be considered for use in an unpredictable situation. The body will resort to ingrained and familiar movements when it is presented with that scenario. The greater the versatility — the more choices the body will have in an unpredictable environment. The greater the efficiency, the greater the chance the athlete will be successful in that unpredictable state. That is the biggest challenge for the athlete. How to successfully deal with that situation over and over again. Keep in mind that unpredictable state will have infinite possibilities. The body needs to be comfortable with this since every situation will be unique to one another.

The first step in the pursuit of versatility is the application of the Champion's Triangle. Prior to practice design one must break down the sport into the scoring skill, transitional skills and hidden habits. A complete understanding of the athlete's functional requirements provides a valuable insight regarding how to achieve versatility for that athlete. From there, one can then correlate and examine the mechanical relationships between the scoring skill, transitional skills and hidden habits. These relationships can be utilized in the formation and execution of movement exercise programs. They can be utilized to improve different facets of sport performance directly and indirectly. Such as increasing mobility, strength, balance, reducing pain and improving efficiency. This provides the athlete, coach, strength trainer and medical professional a multitude of possibilities.

Once the sporting movements have been categorized and examined, the practice design can be manipulated to foster and encourage versatility of motion.

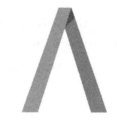

## Practice Design

Practice is the platform for skill acquisition and development. It is the stage where mistakes are embraced and creativity is encouraged. Practice is essential for the evolution and growth of any team or athlete. Without practice, how can one foster skill development?

The Champion's Triangle can be an integral tool in the development of a practice plan or philosophy. It can individualize drills for each player, skill position and athlete. This resource can be utilized from the perspective of the athlete, coach, medical professional and strength trainer.

As I discussed earlier, the athlete loves to practice the scoring skill. If it were up to the athlete, the scoring skill would be the focal point of every practice. However, highly skilled athletes in any sport will understand the importance of the transitional skills they use to compete. They understand that the transitional skills set up the scoring skill. Instead of focusing primarily on the scoring skill, they incorporate transitional skills leading to the scoring skill. For example, a tennis player could practice running to the left before hitting a backhand (right handed player) versus hitting a backhand from a stationary location. These are two different activities. One is artificial — the other is specific to the situation of a game. The body undergoes much different stresses in either case. Emphasizing sport-specific actions within a game-like environment is very effective. This allows the building of transitional skills onto the scoring skill. It enables the athlete to execute the scoring skill with variation.

Variation should be implemented during the execution of the scoring skill. For instance, a volleyball player shouldn't repeatedly practice spiking a ball from the same swinging angle. The athlete should practice spiking at varied angles, heights, directions and speeds. Variation creates versatility. Remember, versatility helps minimize overuse injuries because the body has practiced different forms of motion for the same action. This variation will prepare the athlete for the unexpected. What if, in game, the ball was set farther back than typically practiced? If the athlete has practiced variations with ball location, it typically will not be a stressful situation. However if the athlete has engaged with little variation while spiking, a never-seen-before ball location could lead to a traumatic injury. If the body has not been there before, it may struggle executing the scoring skill at game speed from a foreign angle. If this stress is significant, structural damage may occur.

The athlete must pay attention to hidden habits during a practice session. Performing the scoring skill in the same pattern, direction and speed could predispose the athlete to an overuse injury. The inclusion of the transitional skill while performing the scoring skill encompasses the variability needed to prevent overuse injuries. Incorporating variations in the transitional skill will further develop the overall athlete skill set and minimize the formation of hidden habits.

Coaches understand the importance of the transitional skill from a strategic perspective. Often times their practice plan will primarily focus on the development of the transitional skill. This emphasis is not based on injury prevention but more so skill development and the implementation of the team's strategic play. However, there is danger the practices will exhibit the same flow of motion in a repetitive fashion. This repetitive flow opens up the whole team to possible overuse injury.

I have never understood the use of cones when developing the transitional skills. This is an artificial means of practice. For one, there are never cones on the playing surface during competition. Secondly, this promotes the athlete to have a preconceived notion where to move for a sequence of patterns. In addition, these patterns of movement are never executed in game situations. Instead, the athlete will move according to what is available in the competitive environment. Drills involving cones encourage repetitive motions that are artificial to the competitive setting. Coaches at every level should avoid forcing their athletes into set patterns and movements.

Within practice design, the coach can emphasize the scoring and transitional skills as noted above. However, the important question is how will they be implemented? Now it is important to discuss the type of play and environment that is possible regarding the design of practice. Will the environment and play be fixed or spontaneous? Let me explain the meaning of fixed and spontaneous.

A fixed environment can be explained as rigid, pre-calculated, deliberate and inflexible. A fixed environment yields consistent structural dimensions, no weather influence or significant variance of playing surface. A fixed sport environment will present with standardized playing dimensions and typically be indoors. Weather will not be a factor during the game of play.

Fixed play is usually an individual sport. The play is usually pre-calculated, precise and detail orientated. If we apply this to gameplay, the athlete will have no or little direct contact with teammates or the opponents' movement patterns.

Spontaneous play can be individual, but most times it consists of team play. There is direct contact between teammates and the opponent. Often times specific team systems are implemented but most movement is spontaneous, unpredictable and variable in nature. A spontaneous environment can have varied dimensions, possibly impacted by weather and different playing surfaces.

There are four different combinations regarding the style of play and the environment.

- Fixed play/fixed environment
- Fixed play/spontaneous environment
- Spontaneous play/fixed environment
- Spontaneous play/spontaneous environment

Let's look at all four in detail.

**Fixed play/fixed environment** encompasses play that is not directly influenced by an opponent's actions or movements. The athlete is aware of the routine that needs to be completed and will not change during execution. It is set. The athlete determines the timing and speed of motion. The athlete has complete control. The same can be said about the environment. It is sterile, meaning there is minimal variation in set up. There is minimal influence by factors such as play, weather or actual structural design. An example would be gymnastics. I understand no two gyms are identical, however, when going from one gym to another there will be consistency regarding an event setup and isn't influenced or changed as play occurs. There can be stoppages during competition at which point equipment adjustments can be made to ensure everyone is competing within the same environment.

Another example is Olympic weightlifting. The athlete understands and has practiced extensively specific techniques. No outside influence will affect the style or quality during execution. The environment will also be fixed as the bar, platform and weights are standardized between athletes. The opponent, weather or structural variation of the venue will not influence the skill execution. It is fairly easy to execute authentic practice for the fixed play/fixed environment scenario. The athlete simply practices the desired routine in a setting that replicates the competitive environment.

**Fixed play/spontaneous environment** encompasses play that is rigid and deliberate while competing in an environment that changes — possibly influencing the execution of play. An example would be competitive golf. The golf swing is executed when and how fast the player desires. The athlete is in complete control. However the environment is spontaneous. The golf swing will not be influenced by the opponent, but rather by the environment. The course conditions could be wet or dry. No two courses have the exact same design so a player will be competing on a different terrain every tournament. The weather can be anything from raining and windy to hot and dry. Even the playing surface can be varied. A hilly course will present different types of lies versus a flat layout. A wet course presents different challenges than a dry course because it challenges balance during skill execution. The coach could encourage practice in different weather and course conditions listed above with various lies. This would combine the spontaneity of the weather and unpredictable course terrain.

Swimming would be another example. Before a race begins, the athlete knows exactly what stroke will be executed during the race and roughly the time it will be completed in. You would think the environment would be fixed, but there are several influences that can vary from facility to facility. For instance there is pool depth. A shallow pool will present with more water movement, which can impact a swimmer's rhythm. Any swimming stroke is characterized by execution in a repetitive rhythmical pattern. The athlete strives to attain and maintain that rhythm throughout each race. This rhythm will be the most efficient movement pattern for that swimmer. The water movement within the pool is spontaneous and unpredictable and can impact the athlete's ability to maintain the desired rhythm during stroke execution. Lines at the bottom of the pool are another factor. A swimmer can utilize this landmark determining the timing and execution of a flip turn. Different pool depths will produce different perceptions and can affect a swimmer's judgment of timing and the actual performance of a turn.

Gutters, lane ropes and types of walls at end of the lanes all influence the waves within the pool setting. Again these waves are a threat to maintaining a consistent rhythm of motion. Increasing lane width will yield less choppy water leading to a more efficient repetitive pattern. Swimming outside brings in weather as a possible influence. Suddenly wind and rain can impact the athlete's skill execution.

The difficult aspect for the coach is to help prepare the athlete for these spontaneous variations. How is it possible? Swimming in different venues is a possibility, but remember, the athlete strives to develop and easily reproduce the stroke rhythm and cadence. This would be typically achieved within a consistent environment. Swimming in different settings may just not be possible because of availability or cost. The challenge for the coach is to expose the athlete to variations of these factors so the swimming stroke can consistently maintain rhythm and cadence under different conditions.

**Spontaneous play/fixed environment** is play characterized by spontaneous, unpredictable and variable motion within a rigid or fixed environment. One example would be basketball. The movement and interaction with an opponent and teammates heavily impact skill execution in basketball. Even the size of the opponent can affect the athlete's skill execution. If a player is playing against a taller opponent, the player has to adjust regarding passing and shooting. Every gym is not the exact same. However, gyms are standardized for professionals, college, high school and junior high. The basket height and ball size is set to a specific height for competitive levels. The actual size of the basketball can be varied for different age groups.

In order to develop spontaneous play the coach can implement a spontaneous atmosphere. Mini games can be implemented with different variations. For example, a basketball scrimmage could limit players to dribbling with the non-dominant hand. Another variation could be the playing environment. I know I just mentioned the environment is rigid and fixed but it still can be manipulated for the sake of practice. The team could practice on a wide but short court or a narrow long setup. Even a diagonal layout or a square outline with one basket at one of the corners is a possibility. People may argue that these court dimensions are not authentic to the game of basketball. They are right. However, these variations will place the athletes in unique situations, therefore fostering new movement pattern development. This variety of movement patterns will foster the growth of skill acquisition in a spontaneous manner. Spontaneous practice will yield a versatile athlete. A versatile athlete can adapt and flourish within a variable and unpredictable environment.

Another example would be badminton. The court and net dimensions are standardized producing a predictable environment. Weather is usually a non-factor as games are played indoors. The play is heavily influenced by the opponent's play and movement capabilities. However there are fewer players on the court versus basketball — and consequently smaller playing dimensions.

Playing games encourages the unpredictable and variable play. However the badminton court dimensions can also be altered for the sake of creativity and development of versatility. A coach may suggest playing on one half or playing with opposite halves. Again, this will better prepare the athlete for spontaneous play, which is multivariable and changeable. Emphasizing the non-dominant side, as in basketball, for racquet use isn't essential because badminton is an asymmetrical sport. Basketball utilizes both hands either for dribbling, passing and layups. It relies heavily on the dominant hand. Badminton can be played individually or with a partner verses basketball, which is always a team lineup. Not only does the athlete learn to interact with opponents, but teammates as well.

**The spontaneous play/spontaneous environment** encompasses unpredictable play within a variable and ever-changing environment. One example would be ice hockey. The play is affected by opponent and teammate interaction — it has a changing environment. Play can be at high speeds presenting a challenging element for the hockey player. This play demands instant and rapid reaction and anticipation on an unstable ice surface. There are different positions in hockey but they all live in an unpredictable and variable world. This is beneficial because practice design can include all player positions. To foster skill development, the implementation of game-like situations would be beneficial. A coach may suggest mini games within different dimensions or different player combinations thus encouraging versatile development. The coach may create an imbalance — 4 verses 3 or 4 verses 2 — presenting a unique situation, thus encouraging creativity and innovation. The strategy could lead to new skill development.

I mentioned earlier the hockey environment is ever changing. The ice surface dimension doesn't change during a game but the texture does. At the beginning of the period the ice is smooth and wet. By the end of the period the skating motion has produced rutted areas and light snow cover on the ice surface. This pattern varies from period to period because the combination of play is infinite and unable to replicate. Often times a team will scrimmage at the end of a practice when the ice is worn and snow covered. This affects puck mobility and overall speed of game. It would be an interesting thought to begin a practice with a scrimmage to play within favorable ice conditions. However, it is important to practice with less than ideal ice surfaces so the athlete is familiar and comfortable with such a setting. The size of the surface can vary significantly regarding width and length. This impacts the interaction between teammates and opponents.

A second example would be soccer. Soccer play is significantly dependent on opponent interaction and teammate cooperation. The player reads and reacts, then acts accordingly. The athlete is in charge of when and how to move, but must also react to an opponent's movement patterns. This play is spontaneous and unpredictable as so much depends not just on individual skill set but team play as well. A coach may emphasize mini games and manipulate field dimensions presenting new situations thus yielding movement and skill development.

Soccer's environment is variable in different ways. The size of the fields can vary regarding length and width plus even slope for drainage. There are different surfaces such as turf or grass — both exhibiting differences on ball and player reaction. Rain, snow, mud or dryness can impact the ball and player movement. It will affect the athletes' ability to generate and control speed and power. This makes it difficult to transition from one speed or direction to the next.

It is a challenge for coaches to recreate an authentic practice setting for an athlete. Sometimes a sport can exhibit a small snapshot of a spontaneous skillset within a fixed environment, or vice versa.

For instance, consider a second baseman in baseball. For the most part, the player's position is fairly fixed. Once the ball leaves the bat, the player will have a good idea exactly where the ball will travel and can act accordingly. Sometimes there are surprises when the ball hits the ground and changes direction unexpectedly, but for the most part, it is fairly predictable where the ball will travel after initial contact. If that second baseman is at second starting a double play, there is uncertainty on how the runner will slide into the bag. This uncertainty is important because it can impact the throw to first base. The slide path of the base runner into second base can heavily influence the throwing motion.

Not all sports perfectly fall into of the four categories described above. However, picking the best match can provide guidance to coaches regarding the type of practice design. This potentially can be an overwhelming process but it doesn't have to be. The athlete and/or the coach can break down all the skills of a sport into either the scoring skill or transitional skills. This will bring awareness to hidden habits. Now if the athlete is performing mainly self-practice, the main emphasis will probably be the scoring skill. However, it would be advantageous if the athlete practiced the scoring skill upon completion of transitional skill variation.

Now you have determined the different scoring and transitional skills plus the type of play and environment. So what's next? There are different variables that can be manipulated while designing and executing a practice plan. These can be combined with the different transitional and scoring skills plus the type of play and environment. Some of these I have introduced briefly in previous examples. They include speed, duration, environment, equipment, participants, specificity and execution. Manipulation of all these variables may not be possible for every sport. This will be dependent on the sport and more than one can be manipulated at a time. However, this will provide strategies to assist you when attempting to emphasize spontaneity in your practice design in a sport specific manner.

Speed within a sport-specific drill or games can be varied in a number of ways. Now for the fixed type of play, technique is usually very specific regarding the technique of execution. Therefore varying speed may not be ideal for this type of play. It would be more appropriate for the spontaneous play type.

Different speeds can be emphasized during practice. Sometimes maybe full speed, half speed or even slower. Often, athletes believe they should always practice at high speeds. However, this strategy may not be successful against a team who is faster. A more successful approach maybe to attack that team with slower speeds or a mixture of speeds. That team may struggle defending against a team that can move with varying speeds of execution or a slower speed altogether.

Manipulating the timing of speed changes for transitional or scoring skills can be very effective. For instance, in soccer the athlete may slow down dribbling drawing an opponent near so a pass can be made to an open teammate. In the same example, the athlete may suddenly increase the dribbling speed therefore creating separation from the opponent allowing a pass, additional ball handling or even a shot to take place.

Speed can be altered during the delivery of a transitional skill. An example would be making a pass in basketball. The athlete is dribbling and jogging at a slower speed but then sends off a very fast pass to an open teammate. The opponent may slowly react to this approach since they are accustomed to the slower dribbling speed. It can catch the opposition off guard, as they are not expecting such a difference in transitional execution speed.

The speed could be varied during the transition from one transitional skill to another transitional skill. An example would be a hockey player skating half speed but then performs a crossover at a high speed and then returns to original pace. Again this can be done to create space between the opponent and teammate so a transitional skill may be completed such as a pass.

The duration of a drill can vary especially for the sport where there are frequent stoppages of play within a game. According to the *Wall Street Journal* article I mentioned previously, an average NFL play lasts between 4-12 seconds. Therefore drill duration could be set up accordingly to mimic these time frames. However, the drills could be longer to create an increased tolerance. This will allow the athlete to successfully contribute to a longer-than-average play during competition.

The duration of a drill can be increased in order to foster active recovery following an explosive expression of a transitional skill. An example of this could be a dribbling exercise in soccer. The athlete could perform the dribbling exercise at high speed and then jog for a certain distance before stopping at the back of the line. Soccer isn't like other sports where there are frequent static rest breaks. Therefore the athlete has to develop an active recovery strategy while remaining on the playing field. The development of this coping mechanism can be incorporated into the practice design.

The duration could be so small in order to emphasize the efficiency of a specific portion of the transitional or scoring skill. Practicing a specific component of the golf backswing could be an example. Since it is such a short time frame, this allows the body to completely focus on the efficiency of that moment. This strategy can be used for fixed and spontaneous play.

The environment could be varied in a multitude of ways. Practicing sport outdoors versus indoors brings in the element of weather. Different weather conditions pose different challenges. Wind and wet surfaces could both challenge balance but in different ways. The wind can physically move the body's centre of mass outside the base of support. Rain or snow could produce a wet playing surface. This could alter the stability of base of support therefore causing a loss of balance as the centre of mass falls out of these boundaries.

Different playing surfaces can present with different playing challenges. There may be little traction, too much traction or ever-changing textures. These texture changes present a completely different playing surface compared to the beginning of the game. For example, an ice surface in hockey changes throughout a period. Initially it is very smooth and clean but then transforms to ruts and snow build up. A grass football field can change throughout game play because of wear and tear. At the beginning the grass can provide traction but after repetitive movements, it can become slippery due to breakdown of the surface. Exposing athletes to varied conditions within the playing environment can foster versatility of movement. However, safety must be considered since some conditions could be dangerous.

The environment can also include structural boundaries such as hockey boards, hockey or soccer nets or badminton and basketball nets. The practice setup can emphasize these components or eliminate them. Changing the playing dimensions within the field of play can do this. This can be varied regarding design or size, depending on the playing environment. What this will do is foster innovative and creative play in a spontaneous manner. Since the surroundings would be unfamiliar, this would facilitate variation and creativity within transitional and scoring skills.

Variations of equipment can be carefully altered to improve the efficiency of the scoring and transitional skills. Not all equipment can be manipulated because of rules and safety policies. However for the sake of practice, variations or simple modifications can be introduced. Let us look at the sport of golf. An athlete could practice the golf swing with a heavier or lighter club in an attempt to increase swing speed. The thought behind these two strategies is the heavier club will strengthen the body allowing increased swing speeds. The lighter club will just allow the body to swing faster allowing the body to practice at this speed.

During a hockey mini game a tennis ball could replace the puck. The tennis ball is lighter and bounces. This will be challenging for the transitional skill of passing, receiving a pass or stickhandling because it will react differently to the playing surface and playing contact. The bouncing characteristic can foster the scoring skill of batting the puck out of mid air.

Altering the variable of participants can be done with reference to the number and size. Placing the athlete in different formations will change the space available to function. For instance a basketball mini game could be 4 vs. 2, 3 vs. 3, 2 vs. 4 or 5 vs. 4. The smaller number of participants means there's more space to those who are playing. Also, if the teams are also uneven regarding number wise, the player must be innovative regarding skill execution especially if there are more defenders than offensive players.

Athletes of different age groups and sizes practicing together can vary the amount of water motion between swimming lanes. This adjustment can foster versatility of the swimming stroke because it will function within the unpredictable environment of water motion. This motion will depend on the size and age of the athlete. Older swimmers (to a certain extent) will tend to be faster and more powerful thus creating greater water motion. It is therefore a challenge for the swimmer to replicate an efficient stroke in a variety of surrounding water conditions.

For contact sports, it may not be wise to vary different age groups or sizes due to the possibility of traumatic injury occurring as a result of the physical discrepancies between competitors.

The practice design can focus on specificity. This could be further explained by isolating the development of a specific transitional or scoring skill. In a soccer drill, the athlete may be required to shoot only with the non-dominant foot. This will force the development of the non-dominant side. The athlete will tend to favour what is comfortable and established regarding skill execution. Another example is during a basketball mini game the players are only allowed to pass with a two hand overhead technique. These adjustments can be tailored specifically for each athlete. This can be strategically based upon whatever their physical tendencies and limitations may be.

Specificity can also pertain to a sequence of events functioning simultaneously or built upon one another. A hockey player could be skating, stickhandling and performing the occasional crossover while varying direction and speed. Since hockey is spontaneous play it is impossible to build one sequence upon another because the possibilities are infinite. However, if the athlete is able to execute multiple transitional skills in numerous combinations, then that athlete can string together several transitional skill sequences in response to the spontaneous play. The only time deliberate practice with specific sequence of a transitional skill is authentic is for fixed play. If we look at competitive weightlifting, there is a specific series of actions that takes place during the execution of the scoring skill. It is essential that these actions get completed in a pre-determined order and with a certain speed.

Execution of the skill set can be varied either by performing the skill in an abbreviated or exaggerated means. For example a hockey player may practice an abbreviated or an exaggerated skating stride while stickhandling. This prepares the athlete for a spontaneous, unpredictable situation where an adjustment is indicated and needed.

I am hoping with these examples you envision the endless or infinite possibilities. These variables can be manipulated according to a specific sport, team and player's skill development requirements. This type of detail focus will foster individual and team skill development inadvertently enhancing the overall health of the athlete to withstand the spontaneous and repetitive physical stresses of sport.

If the coach is designing the practice, then the transitional and scoring skills must be established including the style of play and game environment. This will provide a framework whether spontaneous or rigid guidelines need to be implemented during the design. Once established, the design of the practice can emphasize movement variation within the scoring skill and transition skills.

This can be designed according to game-specific skill sets executing in sport specific environments. This variation will minimize the formation and impact of the hidden habits. For both the spontaneous and fixed situations it is important the athlete is versatile. Versatility allows the athlete to endure the minimal variation and repetitive tendencies of the fixed play and environment. This will reduce the incidence of an overuse injury. For the spontaneous play and environment, versatility will allow the athlete to successfully react and adapt. Often times non-contact traumatic sport injuries are due to the inability to read and react to the surrounding play and environment.

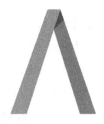

## Prevention of Injury

The increased attention and efforts of offseason workouts, dryland programs and pre-game warm-ups strive to prevent unnecessary sports injuries. Practice during the season should also emphasize prevention of overuse injuries and not just performance enhancement. When I mention practice, I am referring to self-practice, team practice and strength training. This also includes rehab following injury. The Champion's Triangle can help remodel the philosophy of practice providing an opportunity to foster skill development while minimizing the incidence of overuse and traumatic injury.

I mentioned in the practice design chapter there could be fixed or spontaneous play and environments. Regardless of which combination, it is important the athlete practices with variation to create versatility within the skill set. For either a spontaneous play or environment, it is easy to provide an authentic means of practice for that particular sport. Understanding what makes either the play or environment spontaneous is the main challenge. For example, if we look at badminton — the play is spontaneous. Interaction with the opponent provides an unpredictable and infinite type of play. To replicate this during practice, the athlete can simply play a teammate or coach in a simulated game. That teammate or coach can place the shot in different parts of the court. Consequently the athlete's transitional and scoring skill will be practiced in various locations. These various shot locations will organically produce a variety of transitional and scoring skills. For instance, the athlete can be forced to play a smash or a drop shot. Varying the shot location will produce variable transitional skill sequences such as running followed by lunging.

Now, what about a spontaneous environment? The first thing is to identify what categorizes that environment as spontaneous? Is it weather? Is it the type of playing surface? Is it field dimensions? Once that is determined the coach can implement either fixed or spontaneous play within the environment. Maybe practices will include a different environment variation each time — meaning practice during varying weather conditions or switching to different fields.

When accommodating both spontaneous play and environment, it is important practice ensures a variety of transitional and scoring skill involvement. This will not only encourage performance enhancement but also injury prevention. Spontaneous play covering all aspects of the badminton court will naturally produce a variety of sequential transitional skills linked together. This will further develop the physical literacy of the athlete, plus it will develop technical capabilities.

It can be much more challenging to promote versatility in fixed play or environment. For fixed play, the scoring skill is performed in a very deliberate manner. So why is movement versatility important for this type of play? This play predisposes the athlete in developing an overuse injury. Versatility within the fixed play can produce a higher tolerance to repetitive motion and lessen the chance of an overuse injury. Let us take a look at weightlifting. Competitive weightlifting is fixed. The stance, technique and execution are the same with every repetition for each athlete. Over many practice sessions this could lead to injury because it is the same pattern of motion over and over, exhausting the musculoskeletal system. How can it be varied? During practice, vary the foot position or speed of execution. The adjustments do not need to be major to be significant. They just need to be different.

If the environment is fixed, why do we need to change it? Isn't it best to maintain a consistent environment and not disrupt the standard setup? If the goal in practice is creating versatility, the fixed environment can be changed to encourage variation. If we look at badminton, the court's dimensions are fixed from match to match. So how can it be varied? During practice the court dimensions could be altered. For example the court could be broken into half its regular size or diagonal. This would cause the athlete to move in unaccustomed patterns leading to increased physical literacy. Normally the athlete may run and lunge while performing the scoring skill. This sequence may not be possible with a new court dimension. Instead the athlete may adopt a shuffle locomotive pattern that is followed by a lunge.

Monitoring and remodeling the practice of the scoring skill and transitional skills is essential for effective practice. There is a tendency for the athlete to practice the scoring skill in the same pattern, cadence and environment. It needs to be exercised in positions, speeds and patterns of unfamiliarity. These variations can produce new scoring skill patterns and can minimize the formation of unwanted hidden habits and promote a healthy, versatile athlete.

Fostering variation within transitional skill execution can take many forms. It could be a variation of one transitional skill or the variation of different transitional skills built upon one another. The health of the athlete would benefit from as many transitional skill permutations as possible. The Champion's Triangle can make this possible.

The Champion's Triangle can provide structure and organization for such a task. It can categorize all movement patterns for any sport into the three components — scoring skill, transitional skills and hidden habits. From here the athlete, coach, strength trainer and medical professional can examine the structure of play and environment to completely understand what is truly required of the athlete.

The next series of chapters will apply the Champion's Triangle to different sports. First thing to mention is for the sake of chapter lengths; I included few examples in each sport. I didn't dive into excessive detail. Here is why. It is important to note the examples provided are not the only possibilities. These chapters are not meant to be a rigid protocol. Instead, it is meant to be a guide that will help revolutionize practice in sport.

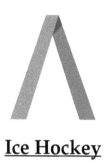

# Ice Hockey

**The scoring skill:** Wrist shot, snap shot, backhand, slap shot and deflections.

**The transitional skills:** Skating, stick handling, crossovers, starting, stopping, turning, passing and body checking.

**Hidden habits (not limited to):** Turning and stopping in the same direction, stick handling same sequence and direction, moving at a consistent speed, get off the bench/climb back into the player's box the same way every time, skating in same direction while circling own end during warm up.

**Play/environment:** spontaneous/spontaneous

## The Athlete's Perspective:

Hockey is a great example of how the athlete loves to dream of practicing the scoring skill. If you watch a pre-game warm-up while the players skate around and shoot on an open net, almost always the puck is directed towards the top corner or just under the crossbar. Why is that? The players have the entire net to shoot at it. Why there? It looks pretty. It changes a great moment into a perfect one. Even if you watch nightly hockey highlights on TV most goals will be scored in the top corner. Even though most goalies will tell you a shot along the ice on the stick side is the hardest shot to save — skaters are always going to dream of the perfect shot. Players won't practice that type of shot because it doesn't look as good as the shot under the crossbar or in the top corner. Remember — creating the iconic moment sports fans crave drives players.

Players love practicing shooting or deflecting. Some players will do so from a stationary position, others while performing a transitional skill. The elite amateur or professional will incorporate transitional skills with the practice of the scoring skill. For example, a player may be skating quickly down the side of the rink and take a shot. As in most sports, there is danger the player will only practice the scoring skill in a comfortable area — only from certain angles and distances. This could lead to an overuse injury.

Hockey players should practice similar patterns that are sport-specific to the playing position. The left-winger will mainly be on left side of ice. Therefore, the left-winger should mainly practice on the left side of the ice. However, it is very important the left-winger will practice from a variety of speeds, distances and angles. For a right defensemen, practicing the shot should be on the right side of the ice, but also further back near the offensive blue line. The shot can go in untouched or be deflected. The defensemen should practice shooting to score and for their teammates to deflect the puck. This is authentic to the position, whereas the winger should practice closer to the net because it is practical for that position.

Each player position consists of different transitional skills. For example, defensemen skate backward more than they skate forward. On the other hand, centres and wingers skate primarily forward. As with all sports, the athlete doesn't typically practice the transitional skills. The elite players realize the value and importance of the transitional skills and will incorporate them while practicing the scoring skill.

There is one way the athlete enjoys practicing the transitioning skills and that is through a scrimmage. Remember, the play and environment for hockey is spontaneous in nature. The most authentic way to replicate such a combination is through scrimmaging. Athletes enjoy scrimmage because it allows the execution of the scoring skill and they are allowed to dream. No two scrimmages are ever the same and some adjustments could be made to ensure further variability. Adjustments can be made to change things up, such as varying playing dimensions or number of players on the ice surface.

## The Coach's Perspective:

Hockey coaches will place a great emphasis on practicing the scoring skills. However, sometimes the scoring skill is executed in an artificial manner. For instance, shooting after skating in a straight line or from a stationary position. Hockey is rarely performed strictly in these two scenarios.

One thing coaches tend to overlook is the execution of the scoring skill for the benefit of their goaltenders. While making a save, the goalie requires sufficient time to execute the skill. However, many times a coach will design a shooting drill that doesn't allow the goaltender enough time to properly perform the save. As a result, the goaltender will move in unintentional ways worrying about the next shot thus affecting the quality of their play.

The hockey coach places heavy emphasis on the transitional skills. All drills will not only encompass transitional skills but also do so in specific patterns. Coaches will implement their offensive and defensive systems with the transitional skills. There is a danger to this philosophy. The players will move in repetitive patterns, predisposing them to an overuse injury. Also this type of practice 'programs' the players to move together in specific patterns of motion. This neglects spontaneity. Meaning the player reading and reacting to an opponent's unpredictable movement pattern. Coaches may include players playing as an opponent during a drill, but again, this role is preprogrammed. The downfall is the inability to react when the player is exposed to spontaneous game situations.

Coaches can create those spontaneous situations with scrimmage or game simulation drills. These drills can isolate certain components of game situations in a spontaneous fashion. This allows the coach to target development on certain team aspects. At the same time, the spontaneity will expose the athlete to unpredictable and variable situations. These drills should be implemented at the beginning and at the end of practice. The reason is the ice surface will present differently in these two scenarios. At the beginning of practice, the ice surface is smooth. This makes passing and stick handling easier to execute. Near the end of practice there are ruts and snow covered areas challenging the player to successfully stickhandle and complete a pass. Practicing in these two situations increases the versatility of the athlete's skill set.

The coach can also vary the spontaneous environment by changing the playing surface and the puck. A cement surface and tennis ball could replace this. This requires a different type of locomotive pattern (running) and a ball that bounces much more than a puck. This will facilitate a greater skill set for the scoring and transitional skills.

The coach can have a significant impact on the development of hidden habits. The continuous implementation of systems in a very deliberate controlled environment can create many hidden habits. How the player turns, stops and crosses over can create hidden habits. This can be rectified if the coach includes spontaneous type of practice. This will force the athlete to move in various directions in an impulsive fashion.

## The Strength Trainer/Medical Professional Perspective:

The strength trainer/medical professional will typically not work with the team when they are on the ice. That doesn't mean it can't be done. Usually it is entirely based as a dryland component. A well-designed plan can transfer over effectively to the ice surface.

A plan consisting of movement-specific patterns can enhance the performance of the scoring skill. Land and ice surfaces are completely different regarding how the body moves. However, exercises can be implemented to replicate what is required of the player while performing the scoring skill on the ice. Plus, I think it is valuable the player is encouraged to practice the scoring skill in a different environment such as land. This will allow the athlete to dream during practice and provide variation and versatility hopefully transferring to game situations.

The transitional skills can also be simulated in a dryland setting. It is here where the exercise program must emphasize versatility and variation. This can be done in a game-or position-specific manner. Simulation of game speed, ability to transition different directions and reading and reacting to the environment would be very beneficial.

An exercise program emphasizing variation of the transitional skills would be invaluable regarding the hidden habits. This would help minimize the negative impact or recurrence of these unwanted patterns.

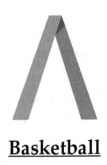

# Basketball

**Scoring skill:** Free throw, jump shot, lay up, hook shot, slam-dunk and tip-ins.

**Transitional skills:** Running, jumping, pivoting, blocking, landing, dribbling and passing.

**Hidden habits (not limited to):** Turning one way, always utilizing the same type of shot, pivoting one direction, taking shots from same angle and/or distance, taking off from same leg, landing on same leg and dribbling with same hand.

**Play/environment:** spontaneous/fixed

## The Athlete's Perspective:

We know why athletes practice the scoring skill — they do it to improve their skill set and to dream of creating unforgettable moments. They love to swish every shot because it adds to the moment. It turns a great moment into a perfect moment. Even though they have the backboard, they tend to not use it because it isn't as pretty as a clean swish. The problem with solely practicing the scoring skill is athletes tend to move in the same patterns or neglect including any transitional skills during shooting practice. This repetitive style of practice can develop hidden habits such as turning or landing the same way and shooting from the same distance, court location and cadence. A suggestion would be to add a couple of transitional skills with each shot and vary the different types of scoring skills and from different distances.

Athletes don't typically enjoy practicing the transitional skills on their own. The reason for this is they don't provide those iconic moments that sport fans crave. The scoring skill does that. However, the athlete should realize developing the transitional skills would improve overall skill set and provide more opportunities to perform the scoring skill. Also, improving the transitional skills will improve the scoring skill because there is some overlap of the mechanics in the skill sets.

In basketball, the play is spontaneous but in a fixed environment. Now the athlete can practice against another player creating numerous opportunities to attempt variation in the scoring skill. An example is one-on-one play. The athlete may have to perform the scoring skill falling to one side or backwards, with a hand in the face or with a change of cadence of delivery. All of these variations will foster versatility in the scoring skill in an authentic manner.

As with most sports there are many hidden habits in basketball. An athlete needs to be aware of the tendencies of their movements and skill sets. Most athletes like to practice what is easy and comfortable. Instead they should practice what is difficult and awkward. This will improve the versatility of their skill set resulting in improved performance and less chance of injury. They must make a conscious effort when they practice to have variation with the transitional skills and scoring skill, as this will minimize the occurrence and impact of the hidden habits.

## The Coach's Perspective:

A coach will understand the importance of practicing the scoring skill because that is how the game is won. The team with the most successful scoring skill wins. However, the coach should ensure when planning a practice that the players perform different variations of the scoring skill at different locations, distances and cadence. Also, performing the scoring skill in game situations (defender attempting to block) will have greater impact on improving the skill set. The reason for this is it will force the athlete to become comfortable when under duress. Meaning it will force the scoring skill to be performed at different angles and comfort levels. The shooter will also like this because they can dream and envision creating that perfect moment.

A coach will understand the transitional skills very well. Remember, the transitional skills set up the scoring skill. You can't have a successful shot without transitional skills such as running, passing and dribbling. One strategy a coach could use to condition the team is to utilize transitional skills as the form of exercise. This will improve the efficiency of the transitional skills and work on cardiovascular endurance. Asking the athletes to repeatedly run lines for conditioning and punishment could lead to injury, as this is a repetitive motion with little variation of movement. This will motivate the athlete to perform during the transitional skills so he/she can execute the scoring skill and create that moment.

The play for basketball is spontaneous in nature. This can be replicated with scrimmages and game-specific drills. This approach creates unpredictable play and impulsive movement patterns. The coach can further variation by manipulating number of players on court at one time or against each other.

Even though the environment is fixed it can still be adjusted to create further variation. For instance, the court dimensions. Scrimmages could take place on a short and wide layout, long and narrow set up or a diagonal boundary. This will force the athlete to discover new movement patterns, therefore fostering a diverse skill set.

A coach can identify the hidden habits for the players on a team. This can be corrected, however, with the design of the practice plan. The practice plan is critical. You can see how it can facilitate the development of the scoring skill, transitional skills, reduction of hidden habits and improve cardiovascular performance. The key is that practice plans are varied and involve spontaneous reaction to an opponent. When athletes determine when to move, they are in control of how they function. When an athlete has to react to an opponent's movement, it is much more difficult because the movement is dictated to them. Emphasizing the latter will develop a much greater skill set in any athlete.

## The Strength Trainer/Medical Professional Perspective:

I will address all three phases of the Champion's Triangle (scoring skill, transitional skills, hidden habits) at once. For all three phases it is essential the medical/strength personnel emphasize variation on every possible level. I am referring to speed, volume, intensity, direction etc. Plus, athletes should have to react to spontaneous situations. If done, this will create versatility of the athlete. This versatility will enable the athlete to repeatedly move in different situations.

The most critical aspect is to emphasize movement when the athlete initiates and when the athlete must read and react to the opponent and environment. This should be carried out in game-like situations.

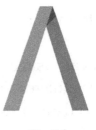

# Golf

**Scoring skill:** golf swing, putting stroke.

**Transitional skills:** walking, running, squatting, lunging, reaching and standing.

**Hidden habits (not limited to):** standing on one leg, same side lunging and reaching, turning head to same side when talking to someone and squatting with same foot position.

**Play/environment:** fixed/spontaneous

## The Athlete's Perspective:

The athlete will want to practice the scoring skill all the time. Golfers do this because they want to improve, but many athletes don't realize the importance of the transitional skills golf. This will lead to a heavy focus on the golfer's scoring skill — the swing. This mindset can be dangerous. It can lead to overuse injury.

Golf is very unique compared to most sports. It is fixed play. The golfer is always in charge of when they move and how they move. There is no influence from teammates or opponents. Most sports are not like that. Another unique aspect of golf is that the equipment is varied for the player to use. The clubs are varied regarding length and weight within the same bag. Hitting balls on the range with different clubs is a good variation to implement compared to hitting the same club over and over. This will vary the movement and swing cadence, therefore fostering versatility for the athlete.

The environment for golf is spontaneous. Each golf course is unique regarding layout and terrain. This will influence the lie of the ball and stance of the golfer. Different weather poses different challenges. Wind and rain can challenge the balance of the athlete. Golfers would be wise to practice with varying lies and weather. It would prepare them for unpredictable and ever-changing conditions.

The athlete must be aware of the hidden habits and pay attention to any repetitive movements or strategies that could impact the overall efficiency of the golf swing. This will be most prevalent when the athlete isn't hitting the ball. Since a round of golf commits a small percentage to the golf swing, the athlete must be aware of what the body is doing in between shots.

## The Coach's Perspective:

The golf coach is the expert regarding analyzing and enhancing the golf swing. They understand the athlete wants to practice the scoring skill repeatedly on the driving range. However, it would be beneficial for coaches to change that mindset of practice. Instead of hitting balls over and over, the coach should try to make the practice less repetitive. Coaches have the ability to break down the swing into different components. Many times they will assign drills emphasizing certain aspects of the scoring skill. This approach would significantly limit the wear and tear on the body and improve swing efficiency at the same time.

The golf coach has a great appreciation regarding the training of the transition skills. However, I would suspect they would leave this area to be addressed by the strength or medical professional. Here is a thought. What if the coach incorporated lunges, walking and squats during range practice? This could simulate the functional requirements on the course. For instance, the athlete hits a driver then walks for a specified time. They would then hit an iron and walk to the putting green. They would finish with a putt or two and walk back to the range to repeat the process. This approach sounds much more authentic than hitting hundreds of balls repeatedly. Also, this is much more logical than hitting fifty drivers in a row during a practice session. You never execute that pattern on the golf course — why practice it?

The coach could suggest practice days when the wind is very strong because this could impact the execution of the scoring skill. If this were practiced enough, the body and scoring skill would adapt. It would adapt and acclimatize to various environmental conditions. Also, the coach could encourage playing on different courses for the exposure of course designs, lies and course management.

The coach can implement strategies to minimize the formation or reinforcement of the hidden habits. For instance during practice rounds, the athlete can be advised to reach and lunge utilizing the left side of the body on odd holes. For even holes they use the right side of the body. Going back to my example how the golfer stands on one leg when waiting for an opponent. This will not change because it is almost a cultural aspect. However the coach could instruct to stand on the right leg for odd holes and left for even. This approach would balance the unilateral stresses imposed by the hidden habits.

## The Strength Trainer/Medical Professional Perspective:

Since Tiger Woods' debut, golf fitness has drastically changed. Training techniques such as squats and lunges are very sport specific in the game of golf. Like I mentioned earlier, in a four-day tournament — excluding practice time and pro-am — a player lunged and reached 288 times. That is a lot over a short time frame. What if the body isn't ready to carry out such a task? Training can prepare the athlete for such physical demands.

There are similar biomechanical movements that occur in the transitional skills compared to the scoring skill or golf swing. For example, walking and swinging a golf club require similar hip motion. If the athlete is walking a hilly course they can consequently develop hip stiffness. This could creep into the execution of the scoring skill, impacting the backswing or follow through. This influence would not only affect performance but also the overall health of the athlete. Therefore, training the transitional skills regularly can help prevent this possibility — in fact, it can improve the efficiency of the golf swing.

Exercise routines must include variation within the transitional skills. Some examples include exercises performed on different slopes, land conditions, weather conditions and fatigue levels. Remember — the body may perform the scoring skill for at least four days straight. It must be acclimatized to this type of workload. If not, the body may break down or compensate, forming a new hidden habit. Exercises must also be performed with speed. A golf swing can attain a speed over 110/mph and then come to rest in seconds. It is critical the body trains generating and absorbing speed. This is very authentic to the scoring skill. The strength trainer/ medical professional can play a significant role in the health of overall performance of this athlete.

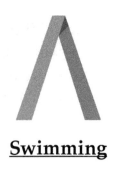

# Swimming

**Scoring skill:** swimming stroke and reaching for wall at race's finish.

**Transitional skills:** start, flip turn and climbing out of pool.

**Hidden habits (not limited to):** turning head to only one side while breathing, starting with same foot in front of other, climbing out pool with same leg leading, hanging onto wall with same hand between sets, open turns to same side, pushing off after a flip turn to the same side resulting in the breakout (first strokes after the underwater portion) and always starting on the same side for back stroke and free style.

**Play/environment:** fixed/spontaneous.

### The Athlete's Perspective:

The athlete enjoys practicing the scoring skill. With swimming it is not just about improving one's performance time, but to experience the swimming rhythm. Competitors have their own stroke and rhythm. The consecutive strokes yield the swimming rhythm. The rhythm is where the athlete is moving in the most efficient manner. Traditionally, swimmers are required to practice large volumes and duration during practice. However the athlete could lose the love of attaining the swimmer's rhythm because of excessive practice. There is danger of not only losing the love of the sport with this style of practice but also developing an overuse injury.

I believe most swimmers enjoy practicing the transitioning skills because they simply want a break from practicing the scoring skill. However, elite athletes will realize how the transitional skills set up the success of the scoring skill. They understand an efficient start leads to a quicker transition to the scoring skill and swimmer's rhythm. An efficient turn creates greater push off from the wall and faster transition to the rhythm of the stroke.

The environment is spontaneous whether it is an indoor or outdoor pool. The athlete will have to perform the scoring skill against the moving water. The water is moving due to all swimmers executing their scoring skill at different speeds and patterns. The pool design can impact the degree of moving water. A shallow pool will experience more moving water than a large pool. Different weather presentations can also affect the moving water within an outdoor pool confines.

Gutters, lane ropes and types of walls at end of the lanes all influence the waves within the pool setting. These waves are a threat to maintaining a consistent rhythm of motion.

The athlete should be able to self-monitor the formation and impact of the hidden habits since the play is fixed. It is fixed and very deliberate in nature. Hidden habits can lead to possible injuries. They can affect the quality of the swimmer's rhythm as well how easily the athlete can get into that rhythm.

## The Coach's Perspective:

The coach is always striving to perfect the athlete's form during practice — especially with the scoring skill. Traditionally, coaches have implemented high volumes of practice with strong emphasis on the scoring skill. Again, a high volume of fixed practice risks an overuse injury. It can be difficult to go against the norm, especially when a philosophy has been adopted for so many years and has become expected. A change of philosophy could emphasize working on the stroke components, transitional skills and the finish.

Another challenge for coaches is creating versatility with a fixed scoring skill. Why does it need to be versatile if it is fixed? The athlete requires this versatility because they are executing the scoring skill within a spontaneous environment. This environment challenges the athlete to maintain the swimmer's rhythm. The versatility is not just for the swimming technique but the ability to maintain the rhythm within a spontaneous sport setting. One solution would be the athletes performing the scoring skill at different pool types. However, this isn't possible for most swimming clubs. The coach could add variation with a staggered start time, mix up age groups and vary athlete combinations. This will result in varied moving water within the pool. This can help the athlete maintain their rhythm within different wave settings.

## The Strength Trainer/Medical Professional Perspective:

Dryland training can play a significant role in the development of the swimmer. Exercises can foster scoring and transitional skill development. A dryland program setup must be functional, sport-specific and non-generic. One reason is that training can influence the shape and size of the body. However, certain body types do not move well within water while performing the swimming stroke. Therefore, it is important the program is tailored for swimming scoring and transitional skills — not simply to build muscle mass.

The dryland program can improve the ability to maintain the swimmer's rhythm. The rhythm is dependent on the body's mobility and ability to transition from one position to another in a repetitive fashion. This transition must be fluid and efficient. This can be trained and it can be enhanced. The athlete's ability to generate speed and power is not dependent on muscle size or isolated contraction. It is dependent on the efficiency of transitioning within the body while executing the stroke.

The repetitive motion of the swimming scoring skill can be dampened by poor mobility and tightness. This tightness will absorb some of the force generated by transitioning within the body. If some of this energy is absorbed, there will be less energy for speed and power. More importantly, this absorption will predispose the body to injury if done repeatedly or in large amounts. Dryland training can prevent this possibility and foster a versatile swimmer within the spontaneous environment.

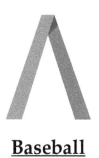

# Baseball

**Scoring skill:** batting, running, diving and sliding.

**Transitional skills:** walking, running, diving, squatting, lunging, throwing, starting, stopping and catching.

**Hidden habits (not limited to):** unlimited, standing on leg more than another, leading with the same leg while sliding or arm when diving, starting with the same leg when running, stepping into a throw the same way, adopting same position when catching a ball.

**Play/environment:** spontaneous/spontaneous.

### The Athlete's Perspective:

Remember it is the skill set that has a direct impact on the outcome of the game — the actions that change the scoreboard. Now I have mentioned several times athletes love to practice the scoring skill, but for baseball I don't believe they love to practice all the scoring skills. It's safe to say that all athletes dream of hitting a home run or grand slam to win a championship. However I seriously doubt the majority of players dream of running around the bases or sliding into home plate. They enjoy hitting. Hitting is performed usually on one side but there are switch hitters. Even if they are switch hitters, one side will typically be favoured more than another. The act of hitting can definitely lead to a physical imbalance of the body and potential injury since it is asymmetrical.

The play is spontaneous but not as much spontaneity as other sports. The one way to add variation to batting practice is to pitch different types of pitches at different speeds and locations. This will alter the location, speed and execution of the scoring skill. This will provide variation in the scoring skill, hopefully creating a more versatile athlete. Baseball is very unique where there are very limited transitional skills leading to the scoring skill. In this instance it would be walking and then setting into the batting stance.

In this sport I believe most athletes will practice catching and throwing more often compared to the remaining transitional skills. The danger is the amount of throwing and catching, and how it is done. If they repetitively throw from the same distance, trajectory, velocity and speed of execution there is a risk of developing an overuse injury. If players never include a transitional skill leading to the throwing motion it will never be authentic to a game situation. It is artificial. If it is artificial, it won't properly prepare the athlete for authentic game situations.

The opportunities for hidden habits in baseball are truly endless. Do they stand on one leg more than another while waiting between plays? Do they lead with the same leg or leg when diving or sliding? Do they adopt the same position when catching a ball? The athlete must be aware of how they lead up to or transition out of any skill set because there are infinite hidden habit possibilities.

## <u>The Coach's Perspective:</u>

Baseball is a very favourable sport for a coach to introduce and develop skills because of the nature of play. There are stoppages in between each play and it is relatively easy to recreate game-specific situations for the scoring skill and transitional skill. If we look at hitting, it is easy to work on hitting specific pitches with different speeds and locations. It is also simple to work on catching balls at different speeds or trajectories by fielding ground balls and pop flies. On the other hand, it is also easy to work on successive transitional skills that occur during a play. For example, fielding a ground ball after running then catching the ball, stopping, turning and then throwing. These are a series of transitional skills that run together and typically are common in a baseball play. It is easy to anticipate what transitional skills and what order are needed to execute a play. However, as a coach, it is very important to vary not the sequential order of transitional skills but how each is performed. Meaning the speed of execution, how it is performed and speed of transition from one transitional skill to another.

The environment is spontaneous in nature. The dimensions of the field can be different from field to field. The shape of the field and walls can also vary. Weather can also provide unpredictable and ever changing conditions. Therefore practice within these varied elements would be beneficial.

The coach must also be aware of the endless possibilities for the development of the hidden habits. Once they are noted, a strategy must be implemented to counteract the possible adverse effects. For instance, when a player catches a ball is the right leg always forward? If so, make a conscious effort to catch a ball with different foot locations.

## The Strength Trainer/Medical Professional Perspective:

One of the biggest challenges is developing a versatile skillset that can be executed following long periods of static positioning. There are so many stoppages in plays and instances where a player is not part of the play. During these periods the athlete will expose and depend on the hidden habits. The strength trainer/medical professional must make note of these habits and then incorporate movement exercises to either eliminate the hidden habit or provide versatility for that action. For instance, if it is noted an outfielder likes to stand with most of weight on one side of body — it needs to be addressed. Since there are so many stoppages in play it is difficult to completely eliminate this hidden habit. Multidirectional lunging exercises, during dryland training, can be implemented stressing both legs in a loaded position hopefully minimizing the effects of the hidden habit. Also maybe implementing a strategy where the player tries to switch the weight shift to the other side after a minute would be effective. A movement program is needed to address hitting (scoring skill) biomechanics with varied paths of motion and speed. This will increase versatility of the swinging motion to handle the variety of pitches a batter may face.

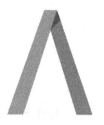

# Soccer

**Scoring skill:** shooting, volleying and heading a ball.

**Transitional skills:** running, walking, dribbling, lunging, stopping, starting, turning, jumping, diving, passing, trapping, throw-ins and kicking in midair (bicycle kick).

**Hidden habits (not limited to):** dribbling, passing and shooting with the same foot — turning and lunging the same direction.

**Play/environment:** spontaneous/spontaneous.

## The Athlete's Perspective:

One unique aspect of soccer is that the scoring skill can be executed when the opponent has to remain still. For instance, during a penalty shot or towards the wall of a direct free kick. Otherwise the scoring skill is usually performed with a transitional skill such as running or changing direction. Soccer players tend to practice the scoring skill with their dominant leg. This can lead to an overuse injury for both legs. One leg because it is repetitively swinging in a relatively same path and amplitude. The other leg is also susceptible to injury because it is repetitively absorbing the weight of the body during the kicking motion. Athletes should practice the scoring skill with both feet. They should do so with different speed and amplitude of execution. Also, altering the swing path of the leg while shooting can place different spins on the ball.

The play and environment for soccer are both spontaneous in nature. Dribbling is often performed amid a cone sequence. This is too artificial. This path is typically not a common pattern during a game. Plus, there are never cones on the field of play — why practice with them? Dribbling paths are typically random and multidirectional. Therefore, it is important to emphasize dribbling drills in a spontaneous environment amongst teammates or opponents. This is much more authentic to the sport of soccer.

The athlete must make a conscious effort to add variation to shooting by switching feet, amplitude, execution speed and swinging path of shooting leg.

## The Coach's Perspective:

The coach understands the importance of implementing and playing within a disciplined offensive and defensive system. The danger of practicing within these systems is that the athlete will be performing the transitional skills in a deliberate and controlled manner. If the practice is too repetitive in pattern of motion, this could lead to an overuse injury. Plus it is artificial to the nature of the sport.

The coach can create a spontaneous environment by utilizing mini games or emphasizing imbalanced teams (number wise). Only allowing one touch per player or only using the non-dominant foot. The coach should further reiterate the importance of practicing variations of the scoring skill. They should also push the athlete to practice their scoring skills from a series of transitional skills. This is very authentic to the game of soccer, plus it will allow the athlete to enjoy performing the scoring skill while developing the transitional skills.

## The Strength Trainer/Medical Professional Perspective:

Since the game of soccer is played within an environment of spontaneity, it is important the athlete develops the ability to transition. Transitioning from direction-to-direction, leg-to-leg and at different speeds. An exercise program should include single leg loading. This is a very common strategy during soccer with shooting, dribbling and passing. This has to be done repeatedly throughout the game in an unpredictable fashion. The exercise program should focus on fostering versatility and efficiency with transition of movement with single leg loading as well. This will not only enhance performance, but also minimize the chance of the hidden habits forming and leading to chronic injury.

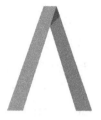

# American/Canadian Football

**Scoring skill:** Running with ball into end zone, reaching over the goal line, kicking ball between uprights, leaping over goal line with ball, diving over goal line with ball, tackling (when opponent is in own end zone with ball-safety), catching ball in end zone, picking up ball from ground (in end zone), throwing ball in end zone and teammate catches.

**Transitional skills:** Running, jumping, starting, stopping, pivoting, landing, squatting, lunging, diving, tackling, leaping, bending down to pick up ball and reaching.

**Hidden habits (not limited to):** leading with same leg when running and lunging, jumping and landing with same foot position, starting and stopping with same leg, using same takeoff leg for diving and tackling, leaning on same leg waiting for next play and sitting in same posture on bench waiting for next possession.

**Play/environment:** spontaneous/spontaneous.

## The Athlete's Perspective:

Football is quite a unique sport — there are numerous scoring skills and player positions. Plus, each position encompasses such a different skill set from the others. Scoring requires the ball to cross over the opponent's goal line or sailing through the uprights. From our list, there are only a few scoring skills I believe may consist of excess practice. That is the running, kicking or throwing motion. Otherwise the remaining scoring skills I believe will be practiced in a lighter volume.

I believe the throwing motion could be the most susceptible to an overuse injury due to poor practice design. This is due to the simple fact that the quarterback will perform many repetitions during practice. The reason for the large volume is because there are so many teammates that have to work with the quarterback on timing. Timing between the quarterback throwing and the different receivers catching. The offensive plays are very deliberate regarding the receiver routes and release time of the quarterback.

The kicker also is prone to overuse injury because the scoring skill is very rigid and deliberate. The kicking motion will be very similar with every repetition. It is difficult to include variability within the kicking motion because it is fixed. However, the kicker could include variability within the transitional skills, which can transfer over to the scoring skill.

There are infinite possibilities regarding hidden habits. This is the athlete's biggest challenge since there is so much downtime between plays. How does one prevent these habits? The athlete will be on the sidelines sitting, standing or walking — always waiting for the next moment. What if an offensive lineman has been sitting for 15 minutes and then in a flash he is expected to produce a very explosive movement against a large opponent? The hidden habits need to be addressed from a preventative and treatment approach regardless of position.

## The Coach's Perspective:

Since football consists of a variety of positions requiring unique skill sets, there are specific coaches for each position. Typically practices are broken up into different positions practicing against teammates. The groups sometimes work individually. However, the coach can set scrimmages where most positions are competing with and against each other. This is authentic because the play is spontaneous. In football, there are infinite possibilities for spontaneous play due to the number and size of the players.

The quarterback could practice throwing the ball running to the left, to the right, forwards, backwards or jumping in the air. This will add versatility to the scoring skill. Throwing the ball at different heights and speeds will add a versatile component for the receiver and defenders.

The environment is also spontaneous since the playing fields can have different slope grades and different playing surfaces. Surfaces could be grass or turf in nature. The weather can also provide variety with different weather conditions. The coach could practice the team on different field types and different weather conditions to emphasize versatility.

## The Strength Trainer/Medical Professional Perspective:

Exercise programs for football need to include heavy loads. Football athletes need to have mass because of significant contact and loading with the opponent. Exercise programs could emphasize a wide variety of movements in multiple directions. This is needed because there are so many transitional and scoring skills in football. Programs could be developed specifically for each position. For some positions, such as defensive or offensive lineman, they perform the transitional skills while under load. Meaning against the weight of the opponent. Performing movement exercises against heavy resistance would be authentic for defensive and offensive lineman. However there is a danger of training with a load repeatedly. If the athlete is training against a heavy load in the same pattern and posture repeatedly, an overuse injury can occur. Varying foot position or movement pattern with the load can avoid this possibility.

As for the other positions, they also perform their skill set under load but not as often or as much resistance as the lineman. These positions would benefit from transitioning in different directions and from one transitional skill to another with speed. These varying movements would provide versatility in their spontaneous environment and style of play. These athletes can also train to transition from one position to another and then engage in a load with locomotion.

The biggest challenge will be to design a program addressing the challenges of waiting on the sidelines between plays. Each player will spend most of the game waiting to play. Typically, this waiting involves prolonged standing, sitting or intermittent walking. The prolonged positioning predisposes the athlete to overuse injury or a traumatic injury. For instance, an offensive lineman sitting for a long duration is then needed to run into the game and engage against a very strong opponent in a loaded position. If a body part is stiff from sitting or standing and then explodes under load, it could tear or rupture.

An overuse injury could occur as well if that player adopts the same posture in sitting or standing repeatedly. These hidden habits place excessive stress on the tissues and joints. They become overused with this repetitive posture possibly leading to an injury.

Training with emphasis on transitioning from one position to another incorporating load will improve versatility. However, this simply may not be enough. The reason is the challenge of the hidden habits forming on the sideline. This issue needs to be addressed, or else athletes will continue to get hurt. I don't know the right answer, but I do know the action time in football is very low. Strategies need to be put in place to reduce these hidden habits. If done properly, I believe there would be a significant reduction in overuse and traumatic injuries.

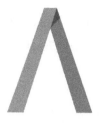

# Tennis

**Scoring skill:** forehand, backhand, drop shot, lob, overhead serve, overhead smash and volley.

**Transitional skill:** running, stopping, starting, pivoting, jumping, landing, diving, walking, and standing.

**Hidden habits (not limited to):** leading with same leg when running, leading with upper body verses pelvis when lunging forward, same foot position when executing one scoring skill and leading with same leg when stopping.

**Play/environment:** spontaneous/spontaneous.

### The Athlete's Perspective:

Most times these scoring skills will be practiced following one or a series of transitional skills. However, they can also be executed in a relatively stationary position. Now, because the racquet is primarily held in one hand, the scoring skill will be consistently asymmetrical. This asymmetry predisposes the athlete to an overuse injury with repetitive practice. It is beneficial to the health of the athlete that a different series of scoring skills occur during game and practice scenarios. The athlete can then practice all scoring skills to provide variation within practice. This variation will enhance the versatility of the athlete.

One strategy to foster versatility while practicing the scoring skill is emphasizing the athlete's shot speeds, locations and racquet swing paths. This would encourage versatility while fostering skill growth.

All scoring skills are based upon a transitional skill. Even the overhead serve follows this rule, as it stems from standing in one position. It is important the athlete incorporates a variation with all transitional skills. These are performed at different speeds, directions, heights and starting points. The efficiency of transition will be critical in successfully setting up the scoring skill.

The play and environment are both spontaneous in nature. It is important the athlete practices in spontaneity — meaning different playing surfaces and weather conditions. These variations affect the spontaneity, plus they challenge the ability to successfully execute the scoring and transitional skills successfully.

Due to the asymmetrical nature of the scoring skill and frequent stoppages in play, the athlete is prone to developing hidden habits. It is important for the athlete to practice a variety of scoring skills off of the transitional skills to ensure versatility and variation of movement.

## The Coach's Perspective:

The ability to transition efficiently is essential prior to the execution of the scoring skill. This process is very influential in the success of the scoring skill due to the speed of the game. Some of these shots are travelling well over 100 miles per hour. Also, transitioning in an efficient and fluid manner following the scoring skill allows the athlete to prepare properly for the next scoring skill. Since the play is spontaneous, the transition will be critical to accommodate the infinite possibilities of play. The coach could set up practice that is based on spontaneity, emphasizing the transition from transitional skill to scoring skill and back again. This type of practice should cover the full court preparing the athlete for as many situations as possible.

The coach can manipulate speed and direction of motion, further increasing the variation of practice. These changes can naturally vary the cadence and swing path of the racquet. This further progresses the versatility of the athlete.

The coach should encourage game-specific practice on different court types and weather conditions. Since there are numerous play stoppages within a match, this can be included within practice, further emphasizing game-like situations.

Practicing with all these variations in a spontaneous fashion minimizes the formation of hidden habits, encouraging versatility of motion.

## The Strength Trainer/Medical Professional Perspective:

Exercise programs should place a strong emphasis on transitioning from one position to another at top speed. This transition should be executed in multiple directions and in multiple sequences. The ability to transition effectively will help offset the risks of an asymmetrical scoring skill.

The program should also emphasize proper weight transfer during transition. This transfer is important because it aids in the implementation of the transitional and scoring skills. Proper weight transfer can be skewed with an asymmetrical scoring skill.

The exercise sequence should last as long as a typical tennis rally. This will further prepare the athlete for authentic game situations. It not only trains the specific movements, but also the energy systems utilized during competition.

Since the scoring skill is asymmetrical, the exercise program could enforce asymmetrical scoring skill movement on the other side. This can help offset the imbalance created by asymmetrical motion.

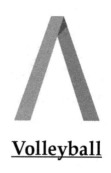

# Volleyball

**Scoring skill:** Serving (overhead and underhand), setting, bump, spike, tip and punching ball.

**Transitional skills:** Shuffling, running, crouching, diving, jumping, reaching, lunging, backpedaling, rolling and landing.

**Hidden habits (not limited to):** Landing on same leg, taking off from same leg, weight shifted to one side in crouch, tipping and punching ball with same hand, diving leading with same hand, rolling in same pattern.

**Play/environment:** spontaneous/fixed. Environment would change to spontaneous for beach volleyball.

## Athlete's Perspective:

Volleyball encompasses a variety of scoring skills. Some of these are underhand, overhead, unilateral and bilateral. The skills most susceptible to an overuse injury in volleyball are the spike and the serve. These are a difficult skill set requiring significant amounts of practice and power. It takes considerable time and repetitions to perform this skill effectively and correctly from a technique perspective. Therefore, the athlete is susceptible simply due to the necessary practice volume for skill development. There is another angle that must be considered. Most times, the athlete will develop a compensatory pattern due to the complexity of the spike and serve. This compensation can eventually produce an overuse injury because it overloads the same area repeatedly.

The entire list of scoring skills can achieve versatility by varying ball location, speed and sport-specific gameplay. The spike is unique to all other scoring skills in volleyball. That skill requires versatility when the body is in midair. Obviously this is a very complex move. Versatility is especially important for the spike because the moving athlete has to adapt to a moving ball while in mid air. The most authentic process to develop this versatility is sport-specific drills or scrimmaging.

The transitional skills for volleyball encompass a wide array of movements. These range from high in the air to low on the ground. The athlete requires versatility of motion in response to the ball traveling at high speeds and changing directions quickly. In addition, the athlete is required to perform these actions among movement and presence of teammates, opponents and equipment pieces such as the net.

There are so many possible hidden habits for volleyball athletes. The hidden habits can be waiting for the ball, initiating movement or landing on the ground. It is important the athlete is well aware of body positioning and tendencies during transitioning and initiating movement.

In volleyball, play is spontaneous in nature and the environment is fixed. The path of the ball heavily influences the athlete's motion. Movement is also influenced by fellow player actions and stationary equipment such as the net. The athlete must read and react to all those variables while executing a skill. One thing unique to this sport is the environment can become spontaneous. Beach volleyball includes both unpredictable and ever-changing factors such as weather and sand. Sand also changes the surface for jumping, landing and transitioning movements. It is difficult to generate both speed and power due to the natural characteristics of sand. As noted in previous chapters, various forms of weather can impact play. In this situation, the flight of the ball and the body's ability to move and react can be altered.

## Coach's Perspective:

The coach needs to help the athlete develop a wide array of scoring and transitional skills. Since the play is spontaneous, the coach can incorporate a variety of mini-games or sport-specific game drills in the fixed environment. This will prepare the athlete for spontaneous movement of the ball, opposition and teammates.

The fixed environment only allows the athlete to use one half since the opponents occupy the other side. This half is also influenced by teammates positioning and transitioning from one position to another. This can be a challenge for the athlete during skill execution since space is limited and ever changing. The fixed environment can be manipulated regarding dimensions of the court or height of the net. Changing the court dimensions for a sport-specific drill will challenge the athlete regarding locomotion and court awareness. This will improve the versatility of the athlete and aid with the infinite combinations of spontaneous play.

Changing net height will alter skill execution of the scoring skill and transitional skills. This does change the authenticity of sport specificity, but does introduce a variation within a fixed environment. This may not be a desirable change for coaches but it is simply an illustration of how the environment can be manipulated in an additional manner.

### Strength Trainer/Med Professional Perspective:

Exercise programs of any type should include movement in the air but also close to the ground. The athlete must be able to perform explosive movement at all heights and angles. The athlete is also required to transition from these heights and angles over and over. This sounds like most other sports, but volleyball is different. Athletes will execute most of these skill sets with the head looking upward. They do so to track and follow the ball. Now the head will lower as the eyes are tracking the descending ball. However, the athlete will perform many actions while looking up. Exercise programs should include the head looking up while transitioning from one position to another.

The transitional skills can be executed in conjunction with a scoring skill. For example, the athlete could be shuffling sideways while performing a spiking motion but not actually hitting the ball. This concept could be applied to and include any volleyball scoring skill, locomotive or movement pattern. You may ask why the athlete would consider this type of exercises? It is to promote versatility. Remember, the spiking motion tends to lead to overuse injuries. If the athlete can perform this sport-specific action in numerous ways, the athlete will be versatile. This will develop a tolerance to repetitive motion.

Exercise programs need to foster versatility at all heights including midair. The athlete will be required to pass or hit the ball from unexpected angles and speed. Therefore it is important the athlete has the physical capability to adjust skill execution very quickly in response to the moving ball, surrounding teammates and opponents as well as the net. This versatility ranges from the athlete in midair to diving on the ground.

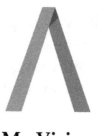

## <u>My Vision</u>

It has been a memorable journey since that Telus Skins Game experience years ago. The Champion's Triangle has evolved so much and I believe it will continue to do so. For so long I wondered why I felt a need to pursue speaking engagements featuring this concept. Why is it important? Why do I keep thinking about it? Why does it keep coming back to me?

I believe it's because the Champion's Triangle is a tool that can identify and prevent overuse injuries in sport, and enhance performance by remodeling the philosophy of practice. As I have immersed myself deeper into this concept, my vision has become much clearer.

I created this concept and wrote this book for you. When I say "you," I mean the athlete, coach, strength trainer and medical professional. This book is not designed to be a set of rigid rules. Instead it is simply a map. I want this map to help guide you and hopefully spark your creative side regarding practice design. You have knowledge and experience within sport. That is valuable and needs to be utilized and fostered.

I believe the Champion's Triangle has the potential to revolutionize practice in sport. However, it can't be done alone. It needs your help. It requires your knowledge and experience. Most of all, it needs your willingness to embrace change and explore new paths regarding practice design. That is not easy to do and the process can be rocky... to say the least. It can be stressful because you are being evaluated regardless of your role. Evaluation is humbling. That's because implementing change can be filled with harsh criticism. Even though most of us involved in youth sport are not primarily working to seek validation or gain recognition. Don't get me wrong, some are but most are not.

So why did I create the Champion's Triangle? I'm hoping it will make practice design easier for you. Because at the end of the day, it is all about helping you foster empowering relationships between athlete and sport that lasts a lifetime.